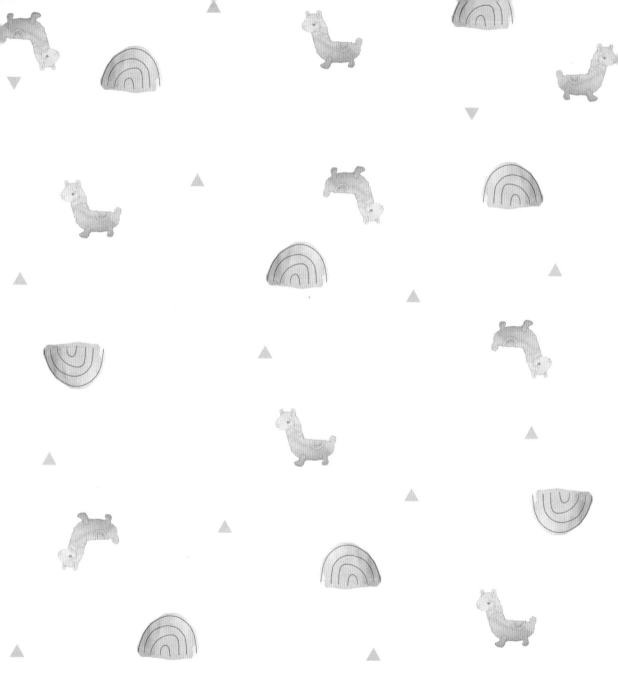

You Got This, Mama!

From Boobs to Blowouts, a Survival Guide for New Mothers

Written and illustrated by
Liz Swenson

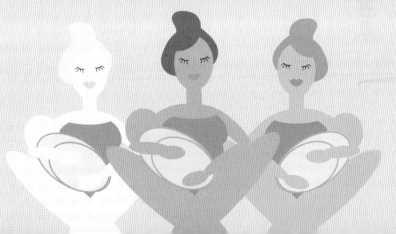

Published by Familius LLC, www.familius.com
1254 Commerce Way, Sanger, CA 93657

Familius books are available at special discounts for bulk purchases, whether for sales promotions
or for family or corporate use. For more information, email orders@familius.com.

Library of Congress Control Number: 2020947679

Print ISBN 9781641704496
Ebook ISBN 9781641705004
KF: 9781641705202
FE: 9781641705400

Printed in China

Edited by Laurie Duersch and Alison Strobel
Cover and book design by Liz Swenson

10 9 8 7 6 5 4 3 2 1

First Edition

BEING A MOM
HAS MADE ME
SO TIRED.
AND SO HAPPY.

Tina Fey

Contents

♡

So the adventure begins...................1

Chapter 1 Poop...................7

Chapter 2 Boobs...................23

Chapter 3 Sleep...................57

Chapter 4 Sanity...................89

Chapter 5 Body...................117

Chapter 6 Sex...................155

Chapter 7 Baby...................173

Acknowledgments...................204

So the
adventure begins

Welcome to being a mama!

This is my humble attempt to give you any and all tidbits I have gathered to help you survive your first baby. You will not only survive, but will thrive and be the most amazing mother because it is in your nature. This guide contains some helpful info on boobs, sleep, poop, and other useful subjects to help you along on this exciting new adventure. You got this!

1

YOU are HERE

NEW BABY!

THIS life is PRETTY AMAZING

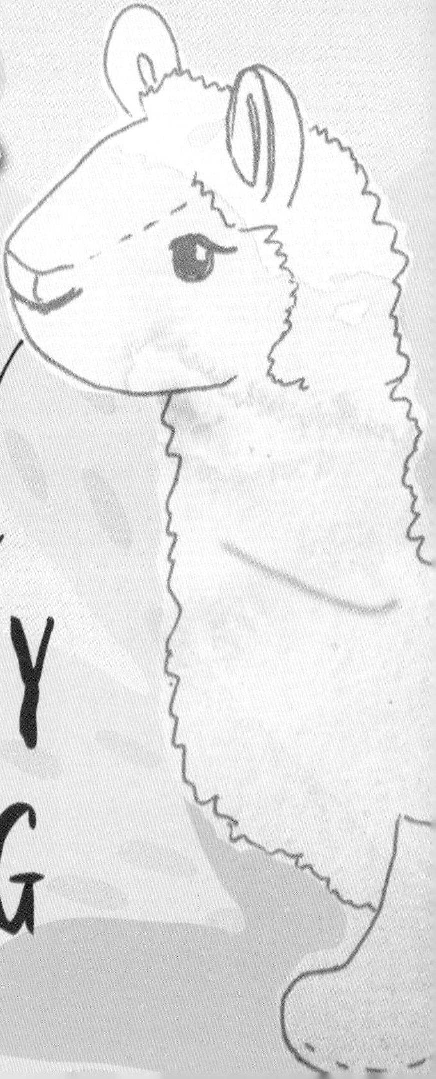

SURVIVING BABY

Here are my 2 rules that have helped me the most:

1. Lower your expectations.

2. Put on your air mask.

ON LOWERING EXPECTATIONS:

Being a mom looks less like Pinterest and more like Picasso.

air mask

/er-mask/

noun

1. The act of taking care of yourself first to be able to care for others.

   "Place the air mask on yourself first before helping small children or others who require assistance."

CHAPTER 1

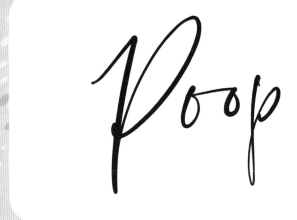

Poop

I'm not going to lie. I have always hated the word "poop." It just grosses me out. I don't like talking about it or even thinking about it, buuuut I'm a mom, so it is now a big part of my life. In the beginning, poop (and pee for that matter) is not only an experience, but a tool. Poop tells you a lot about the health of your baby, and that's your whole wide world now. So poop is important. Pay attention to it, and report anything weird you see. Also, try to dodge it when it's explosive. Welcome to being a mom. You care about poop.

Poop* Progression:

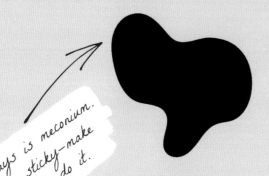

1st Poop: Meconium
Tar/Black

First 2 days is meconium. It's very sticky—make your hubs do it.

2nd Poop:
Green/Yellow & Seedy

3rd Poop:
Yellow

The yellow stuff in the beginning is highly projectile. Be on your toes & ready to act fast when changing those diapers.

These are breastfed colors.

MORE TYPES OF POOP:

HEALTHY

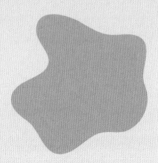

**Peanut butter-like
(formula fed)**

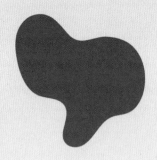

**Dark, smelly, & thick
(solid food)**

You may want to check in with your doctor if you see the following for a couple of days in a row:

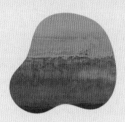

**Slimy & green poop
(allergy or infection)**

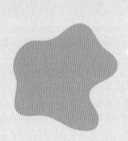

This will dehydrate baby, so give them extra fluids.

**Watery & can come in all colors
(diarrhea)**

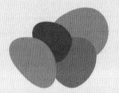

**Hard & pebble-like
(constipation)**

Avocados can help if baby is on solids.

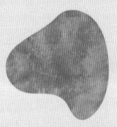

**Frothy & green poop
(baby is not nursing
long enough)**

Try nursing on the same boob you left off on at the next feeding.

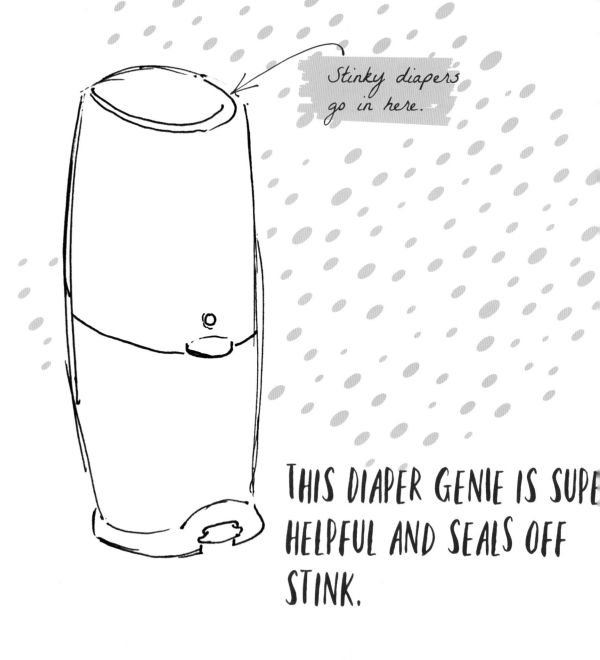

blowout

/ˈblō͜ˌout/

noun

1. When a diaper is so full of poop it ruptures, causing poop to escape from all sides.

   "Oh no! The babe had a blowout and we forgot backup clothes."

Pack the backup clothes in a ziplock bag. This allows you to have a place to put dirty clothes in where they won't leak until you can get home to wash.

THE WAY YOU WIPE MATTERS.

*Place a clean diaper over his penis while you change to prevent surprise pee squirts.

* Make sure to clean under his scrotum.

*As you put on a fresh diaper, point penis down to prevent leaks.

*Always wipe girls from top to bottom.

* Make sure to clean in between the vagina folds.

*During bath time, avoid soap on the vagina—it can cause UTIs.

HOW TO GET BABY POOP OUT OF YOUR JEANS:
(or baby clothes)

Step 1: Rinse off excess poop.

Step 2: Apply dish soap to stain; scrub a little.

Step 3: Lay out in the sun for a bit. *Don't rinse dish soap off.*

Step 4: Wash like normal.

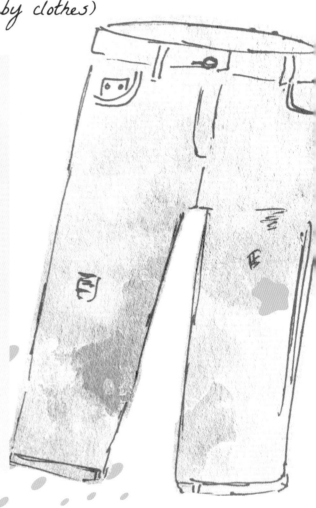

So statistically, you will get
a lot of poop on you.
Hopefully not in your mouth!

FACT:
THE AVERAGE BABY REQUIRES
OVER 2,000 DIAPER CHANGES IN
THEIR 1ST YEAR.

SH** COULD BE WORSE

Keep those expectations low and those gratitudes high!
Yes, there are a variety of bodily fluids on you, but you also happen to have the most perfect thing ever created in your arms.

I'M ALLOWED TO MAKE A BIG DEAL OUT OF THINGS THAT FEEL REALLY BIG TO ME.

Like how many times my baby pooped today.

Anne Carly

This is a MUST once baby starts solid foods. The poopy diapers get SO stinky!

bomb bin

/bäm-bin/

noun

1. A trash bin kept outside, in the garage, or on the porch, used exclusively for poopy diapers so they don't stink up the whole place.

"So glad we have a bomb bin on our porch now that the baby has started eating solids."

CHAPTER 2

Boobs

What a miracle, a joy, and a burden these boobs are. Since junior high they have been changing shape just as we have, and now through this whole baby thing, they are going to undergo their biggest transformation yet. It's downright silly all the things that happen to your boobs through this process. Your boobs will make you laugh, they will 100% make you cry, and you may even witness them sustain a perfect little life for months. But however you feed your baby is perfect. And whatever ends up happening, make sure to give your boobies, and yourself, lots and lots of love and a little bit of slack.

BOOB PROGRESSION

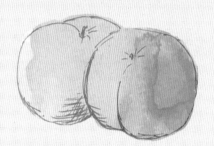

Before baby

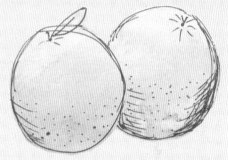

Pregnant

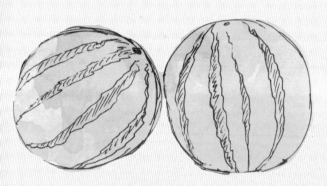

Lactating

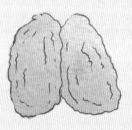

After baby

BREASTFEEDING HURTS

(like, a lot)

I know 1 person (of like 100) who said it didn't. It hurt me for 3 weeks, then got better.

...BUT
IT'S TOTALLY WORTH IT.
(actually one of my favorite parts of momming)

*Take advantage of breastfeeding classes before baby and lactation consultants while in the hospital.

*The gel pads from the hospital are <u>amazing</u>! I've seen them on Amazon too.

Breastfeeding can also not work, & if this happens, don't beat yourself up!...

Today's Goal:

Keep the tiny
human alive

BUT FOR REAL:

DON'T BEAT YOURSELF UP

If breastfeeding doesn't work, or isn't your thing, or just hurts too damn much, the truth is your baby will be just fine. My husband is a full-grown 6'4" adult Viking and he was formula fed.

You got

this.

Babies are born with a powerful suck reflex, but that doesn't mean they know how to latch...and it HURTS when they get it wrong.

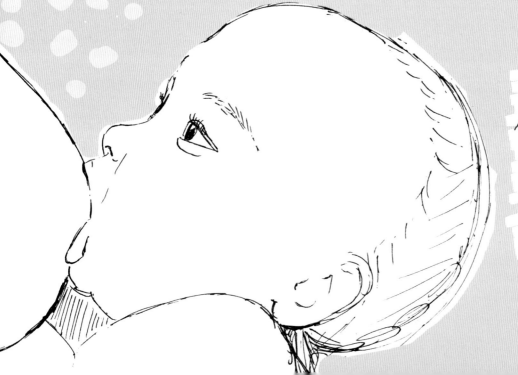

If it's hurting, get in touch with a lactation consultant!

Lower your expectations and mentally prepare yourself for it to be hard. You & baby are learning something new together. ♡

engorgement

/ĕn-gôrj'-ment/

noun

1. When the breast tissue overfills with milk, blood, and other fluids. This causes your breasts to feel very full, to become hard and painful, and your nipples to appear flattened and tight.

   "Wow, frozen peas really do help the engorgement feel better."

An ice pack can help reduce the pain and swelling. Frozen peas are my fave.

Reach out to your people!

Lactation consultants can be super helpful. Ask mama friends or talk with your doctor. You have lots of resources out there.

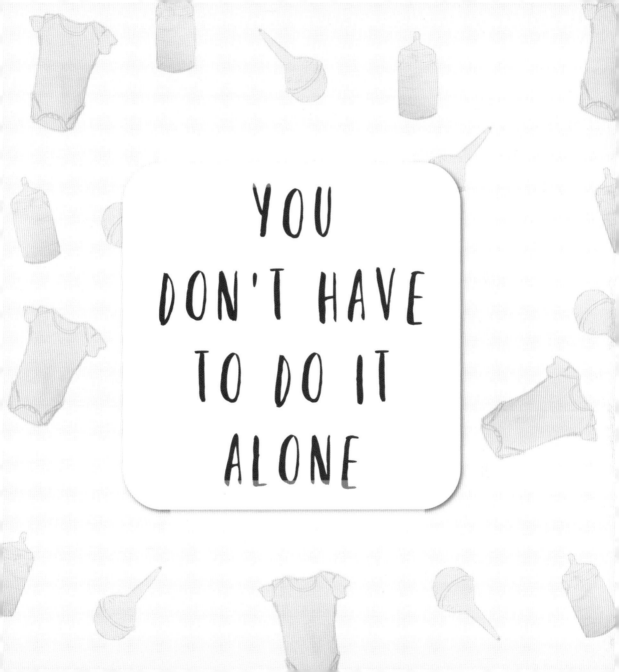

letdown

/let-doun/

noun

1. A milk ejection reflex, in which the hormones released by the pituitary gland cause milk to express from nipples.

   "I wear nipple pads when I grocery shop because if I hear a random baby cry, I'll have a letdown."

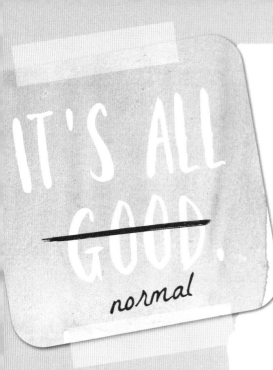

IT'S ALL GOOD.
normal

Letdowns can :

* Hurt (like a tingly, painful squeeze).

* Not hurt.

* Not be noticed at all.

* Happen while your baby is nursing.

* Happen when your baby cries.

* Happen when someone else's baby cries.

* Happen if you just think about your baby.

* Happen when you have an orgasm.

* Not happen while you are trying to pump.

* Not happen while your baby is nursing.

Letdowns are triggered by your hormones. So if you are stressed, tired, or upset, that can change things.

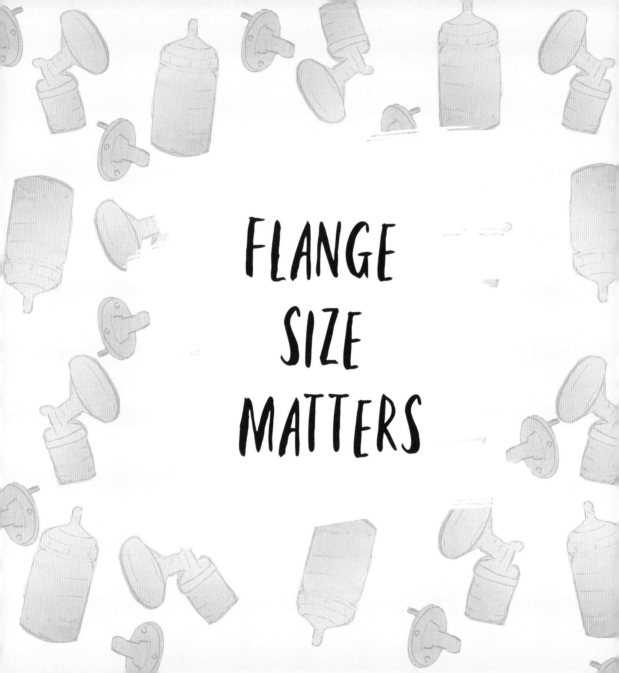

FLANGE
SIZE
MATTERS

I have used many pumps and they were all great. My favorites enabled me to move about my house as needed, but everyone has different needs. What I found most important was that the flange I used fit my nipple properly. Make sure your areola (the soft pigmented skin around the nipple) is not being sucked into the tube.

BOOB LOVE

* Make sure baby has a deep latch. (Work with a lactation consultant if they don't.)

* Gel pads are amazing! (Normally the hospital will give you some.)

* Change nipple pads once they are wet.

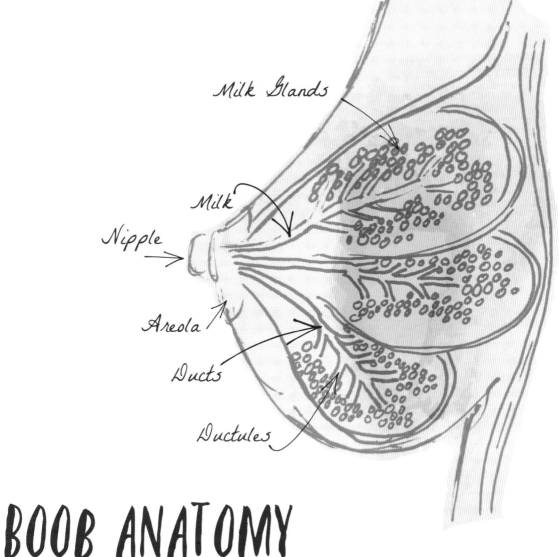

Milk Glands

Milk

Nipple

Areola

Ducts

Ductules

BOOB ANATOMY

Spit-up is normal.

And mostly stops by 6 months.

DRINK SO MUCH WATER, IT'S CRAZY.

I'm not sure
how,
but I will.

Like _mastitis_ or _thrush._

If you have been
nursing for over 3 weeks
and breastfeeding is still
hurting a lot, something
may be wrong. Get in
touch with a lactation
consultant or your doctor.

Anything can happen.

The #1 cause of
mastitis
is stagnant milk.

This feels like: fever, chills, achiness, a sore red spot on your boob.

mastitis

/maˈstīdəs/

noun

1. A painful infection of the breast tissue caused by bacteria that usually occurs in a blocked duct or cracked nipple.

   "Mastitis sucks!"

Ugh, it does so much! If you are an over-producer, this is just one of those things that happens often. You can massage to try and clear the duct, and keep feeding a bunch on the affected boob, but this is a call-the-doctor-right-away thing.

feed (or pump) more frequently => more milk

feed (or pump) less frequently => less milk

Feed on one boob each feeding to reduce supply (this is a mellow version of block-feeding) & use a Haakaa pump while nursing to increase supply.

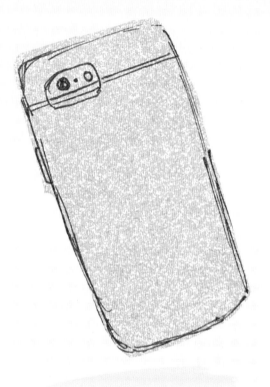

There's an App for That:

-When was the last time you fed your baby?

-Which boob did you use?

-How long did the baby eat?

-How much did the baby eat?

-How many times has the baby pooped in the last 48 hours?

-How long has the baby slept today?

I highly recommend a baby tracker app. You will be so sleep deprived, you can't remember what goes in the fridge or pantry. There are so many awesome free apps that help.

HOW BABIES ASK TO BE FED:

HUNGER CUES

I'D LIKE TO BE FED, PLEASE:

* Licking lips.
* Sticking tongue out.
* Sucking on anything nearby.

IF YOU DON'T FEED ME SOON, I WILL BE HANGRY:

* Rooting (turns head trying to find a nipple).
* Fidgeting, squirming body motions.

HANGRY:

* Crying.
* Red-faced.
* Rapid, jerky body motions.

Ouch!

YOUR BABY MIGHT BITE YOU.

You can teach them not to do it again by waiting about 30 seconds to a minute after they bite to feed again.

NIGHTTIME NURSING BRAS ARE THE BEST!

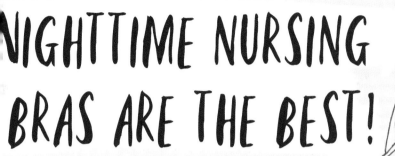

Invest in a couple of good ones. You are basically in your PJ's for the first couple of weeks anyway. I wore mine all day long! They are so comfy and provide quick and easy boob access.

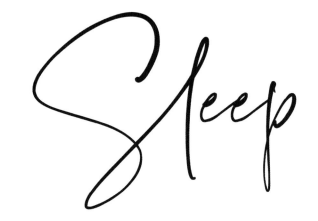

CHAPTER 3

Sleep

Oh, elusive sleep. Here's the thing: no matter what you do, you will be tired. Babies sleep a lot, but not all in one big chunk...at least, not at first. And those late-night feedings disrupt your one big chunk. Getting a baby to sleep so you can sleep becomes a big part of your life. There's a lot of information out in the world on the best way to do this, and you can get really desperate and confused. So I'll keep it simple with everything we did, plus some sleep cheat sheets for all the different ages. Like everything else, go with your gut. Every baby is different, every family is different, and there is no one "right way." Hopefully you will find the following pages helpful and encouraging. We were really lucky it worked great with our boys. As always, keep those expectations low. You will be tired no matter what—you have a new baby! But maybe these tips will help you feel a little less tired than you could be. Good luck!

DON'T WORRY, BE HAPPY.

Said no sleep-deprived person ever.

Wake up
and be
awesome

And if you're
lucky–take a shower!

AN AVERAGE NIGHT IN THE FIRST 6 WEEKS:

Baby cries. -> Dad wakes up, changes her, hands her to Mommy. -> Mommy feeds. -> Hands baby back to Dad to be re-swaddled and put to bed. Repeat.

"I swear I have it all together... I just forgot where I put it."

WARNING

If you haven't gotten REM (requires 4 hours of uninterrupted sleep) in over 4 days, you will become loopy—and by loopy, I mean crying and really angry with your partner.

HOW BABIES ASK TO BE PUT TO SLEEP:

Sleep Cues

*eye rubbing

*staring into space

*being fussy

*yawning

When you see any of these signs, put your baby to sleep as soon as you can. They are ready!

During the day, feed baby => then change diaper.

During the night, change diaper => then feed baby.

TYPES OF SLEEP

	Type of sleep:	What it looks like:
1	Drowsy	Heavy eyelids, long blinks, almost asleep.
2	Light sleep	Baby moves and will startle at noises, and can cry out.
3	Deep sleep	Baby is very still and doesn't move or startle.

GOOD TO KNOW!

SLEEP BEGETS SLEEP

I know, it's a little counterintuitive, but true. Holding off on a nap so that they sleep better at night doesn't work.

SNUGGLES

SWADDLES

SLINGS

Babies like being snuggled up tight, just like in Mommy's tummy. So swaddling can help get baby to sleep and sleep better. Slings and baby carriers can also get a baby to sleep pretty quickly, especially when they are fussy or overtired.

SCHEDULE ~~Patterns~~

SCHEDULE

SCHEDULE

OK, so the word "schedule" is a bit of a stretch for a baby. You can nudge a baby toward patterns that make your life easier and make the baby happier, but you can also drive yourself insane trying to get your baby on an actual schedule—it's a baby, not a train.

PATTERN BUILDING
(MONTHS 1-3)

Here's what I've got:

1. Set a "wake" time (mine is 7am), feed baby right then and every 2.5-3 hours during the day. Yes, you will need to wake a sleeping baby to do this sometimes.

2. After 10pm, let them sleep as long as they want. Don't worry about the 3-hour rule.

3. Avoid sleep aids if at all possible. If not possible, do anything and everything to calm down the screaming baby at 3am.

MONTH 1
(DAYS 0-30)

Basically your baby is going to sleep A LOT this month. Normally, baby will fall asleep right after you feed him. Just feed when they wake up or 2.5 hours after they last ate, whichever comes first, and that's as much as you can hope for as far as a schedule goes.

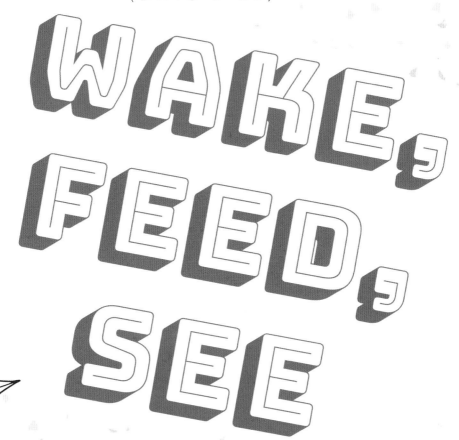

WAKE, FEED, SEE

When your baby wakes up, feed her, and then see if she goes back to sleep or wants to look around for a bit before falling asleep.

FEED,

WAKE,

SLEEP

This is the classic baby mantra, and it's very helpful for creating nice patterns. The idea is when baby wakes up you feed him, let him play awake for a bit, then put your baby to sleep.

MONTH 2

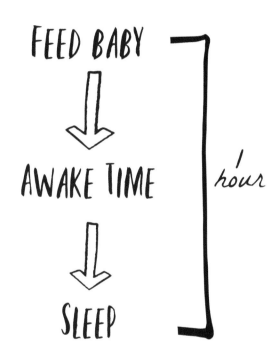

FEED BABY

⬇

AWAKE TIME

⬇

SLEEP

} 1 hour

So if baby wakes at 2:00pm, feed her, and she should be napping at 3:00pm.

MONTH 3
(DAYS 61-90)

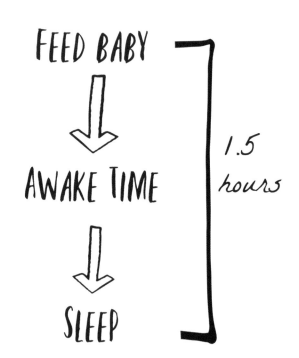

FEED BABY

⬇

AWAKE TIME

⬇

SLEEP

1.5 hours

So if baby wakes at 2:00pm, feed her, and she should be napping at 3:30pm.

MONTHS 4-12

At this point, your baby will (hopefully) be showing some patterns. I've always liked to follow their lead. My babes started going down for their long night sleep around 7pm and would feed once during the night, then eventually not at all. All babies are different, and every night is different. Just try to roll with it and let them sleep when they ask for it during the day.

4 Month Sleep Regression

Ugh...yes, this is a thing. And it's no fun.

REMEMBER THAT YOU ONCE DREAMED OF BEING WHERE YOU ARE NOW.

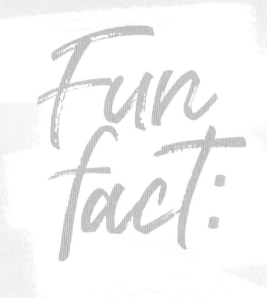

Fun fact:

Babies randomly cry at night, or during a nap. Wait a minute before you get them because they are still sleeping and won't be happy when you get them.

Mobiles & Sound Machines

Actually, super functional and helpful getting your baby to sleep!

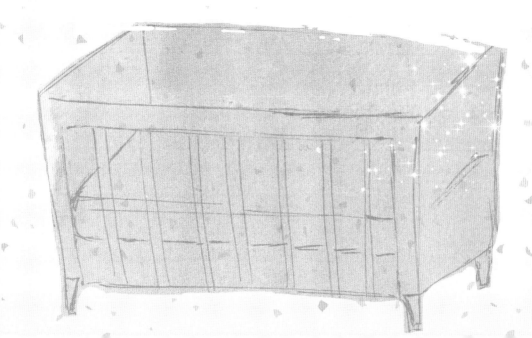

ALL
BITS
ARE
OFF

If your baby i

*Teething.

*Experiencing a
growth spurt.

* Having a
mental leap.

*This applies to both sleep and feedings.

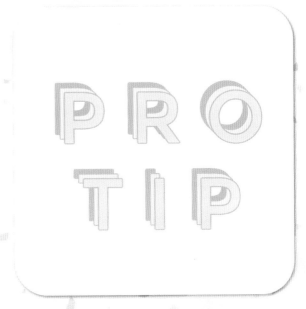

Put your baby to bed sleepy, but awake. It's good for them to learn to chill and sleep on their own. It won't happen often, but it's good to try.

Start each day with a grateful heart.

IF BABY SLEEPS

↓

YOU SLEEP!

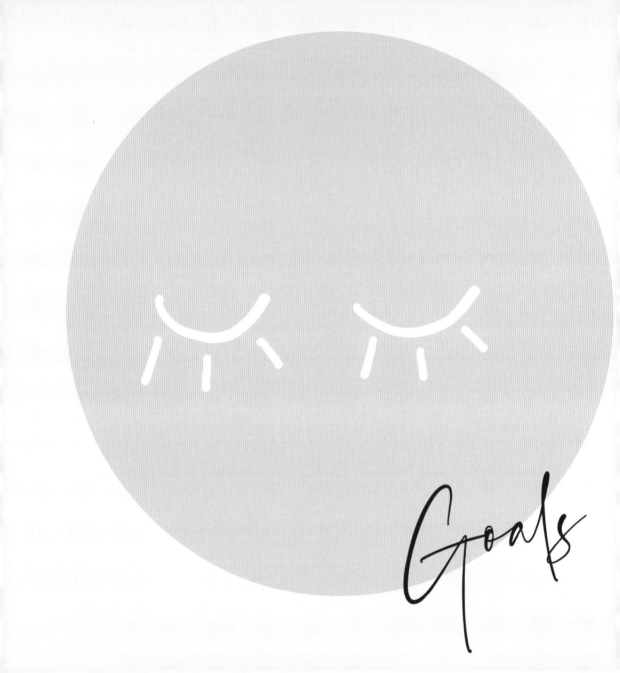

Goals

MAKE A WISH

Let this baby sleep at least 5 hours a night!

CHAPTER 4

Sanity

Oh, Sanity, there has never been a thing on this earth that you have loved like this baby, and it is often overwhelming. Reading too many books about parenting will make you crazy, and so will all the unsolicited advice from your mother, sister-in-law, the cashier checkout lady, or even me. The thing is, being a mom is an intensely personal thing and everyone is trying their best. As you gather information to keep your baby alive (& hopefully happy), keep in mind that YOU know best. If any counsel or recommendations from a book or other people don't feel right, then don't push it. Advice like this should be thought of like a hotel concierge—it can be useful if you are lost or need help, but mostly can be ignored.

This is insanely hard!! But also the best thing ever!

the trenches

/T̲Hə tren(t)SH/

noun

1. The first 3 months with a new baby.

"This too shall pass. We just need to survive the trenches."

Truly though, the first few months are so hard. Give yourself (and your partner) all the breaks.

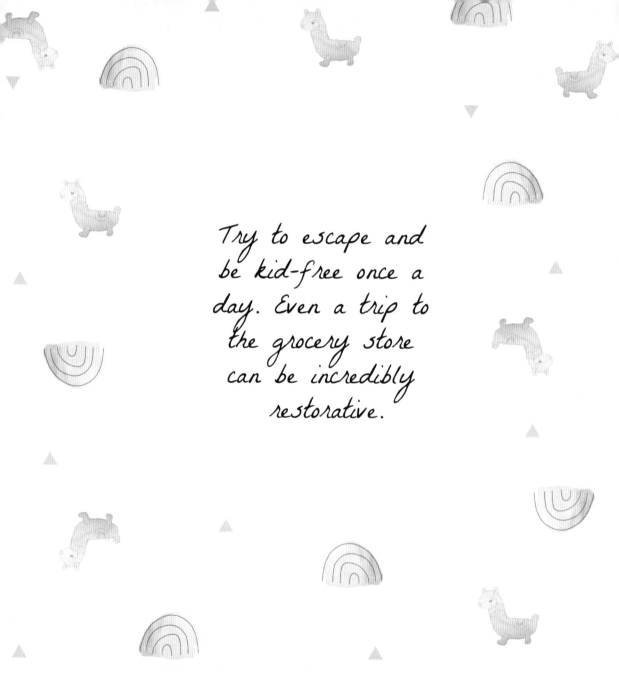

Try to escape and
be kid-free once a
day. Even a trip to
the grocery store
can be incredibly
restorative.

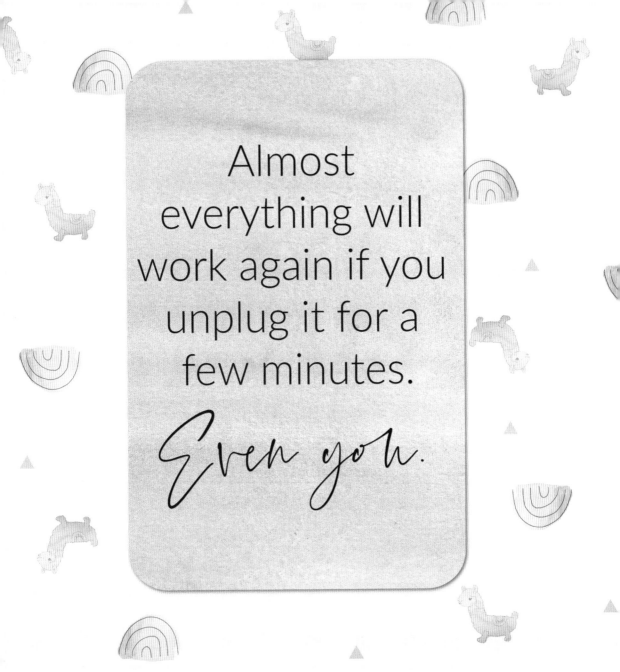

Almost everything will work again if you unplug it for a few minutes.

Even you.

You have
mama
instincts;
I trust them.

BEING A MOM IS LIKE FOLDING
A FITTED SHEET—NO ONE REALLY
KNOWS HOW TO DO IT.

You will be ok.

(AND IT'S OK NOT
TO FEEL OK)

Postpartum depression is real, and OK, and so very common. If you think anything that scares you, speak about it to your doctor, partner, and best friend. It's OK to not be OK.

Stay close to people who feel like sunshine.

Friends that call you
from the grocery
store to see if you
need anything

are the best kind of friends.

ON CRYING:

This will happen a lot.

It doesn't mean anything is wrong and it's super normal. Your body is coursing with hormones. You are sleep deprived. And you are experiencing a new type of stress, the keep-my-baby-alive stress, and it's overwhelming.

CRYING AND LAUGHING ARE YOUR BODY'S PHYSICAL MECHANISMS FOR RELEASING STRESS. SO HAVE A GOOD LAUGH, OR A GOOD CRY, AND TRY TO GET SOME SLEEP. YOU WILL FEEL A LOT BETTER.

Some days, doing "the best we can" may still fall short of what we would like to be able to do. But life isn't perfect—on any front—and doing what we can with what we have is the most we should expect of ourselves or anyone else.

Mr. Rogers

Mistakes
are proof
you are trying.

Plan Ahead

Diaper Bag Checklist
* change of clothes
* extra diapers
* feeding basics
* wipes (so many wipes)
* hand sanitizer
* muslin wrap
* pads for mama

While baby is sleeping, get your diaper bag stocked and ready to go.

* And always re-stock when you get home.

Iced coffee must have been the invention of a mom. At some point, she gave up on trying to have her coffee warm, put ice in it, and called it her new favorite drink.

DO THE BEST YOU CAN UNTIL YOU
KNOW BETTER. THEN WHEN YOU
KNOW BETTER, DO BETTER.

Maya Angelou

Yup, this is pretty much all you can do. Don't beat yourself up along the way. You got this!

"I FEEL LIKE HE'S CONSTANTLY CHALLENGING MY BELIEF THAT I HAVE ANY KIND OF UNDERSTANDING OR CONTROL."

-Me
(when my first baby was 8 weeks old)

Sanity Savers

Avoid the internet at all costs. Find a good book and stick with it. My doctor recommended American Academy of Pediatrics: <u>Caring for Your Baby and Young Child.</u>

*Clean everything with vinegar.

*Muslin swaddles can be used as nursing covers, burp cloths, blankets, or changing pads. I never leave the house without one!

*Invest in a nice outdoor park blanket.

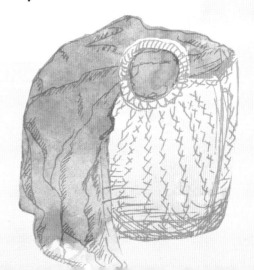

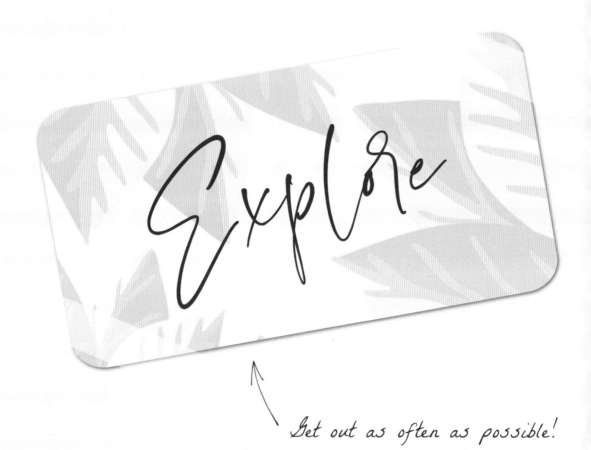

Explore

Get out as often as possible!

Lose your head in the clouds.

Listing things you are grateful for can help you fall asleep on anxious nights.

Everything is figureoutable.

This too shall pass.

And it really will. This impossible, insanely hard moment will pass. Deep breath in, then let it out. I love you—you got this!

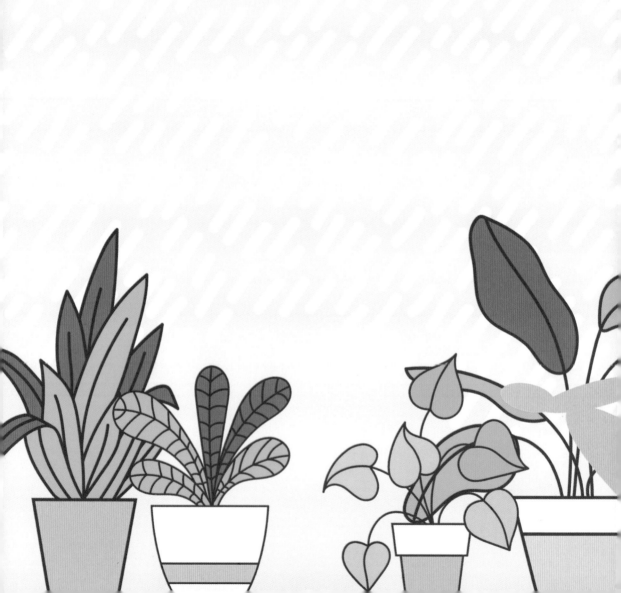

CHAPTER 5

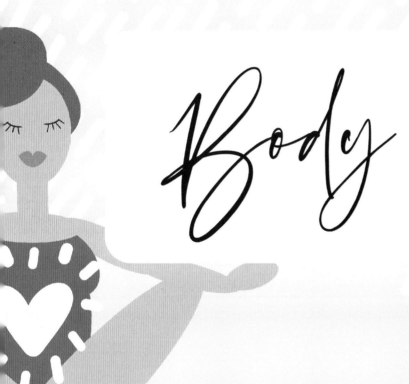

Body

Alright, beautiful. Here's the thing: your body is perfect. Yup, perfect. I think you are the most beautiful you have ever been. I'm in awe of your body's strength and resilience. I'm so grateful you and baby are healthy and you are healing. It's just plain amazing that your body created a life—a tiny, perfect life. Your body may feel different now: your boobs are doing all kinds of crazy things, and your lady parts too. Nourishment is important. Care for your body with the same amount of love you are showering on your little babe because—trust me—you deserve it. The more you love on yourself, the better you will feel, the better you will "mom." Drink lots of water and eat lots of veggies. Your body is amazing mama; never forget it.

You don't need
your body back;
it's been here with
you through it all.

NOURISH YOUR BODY

Nourish it with love, good food, lots of water, long walks, and lots of patience.

Nourishing your body can mean many things. It can mean drinking a green juice every morning (my mom brought me one every day in the hospital and I swear that is part of why I healed so well each time), and it can also mean never restricting yourself. If you are craving donuts, then you should be eating donuts. Your body knows what it needs. Trust it.

SALAD FOR BREAKFAST

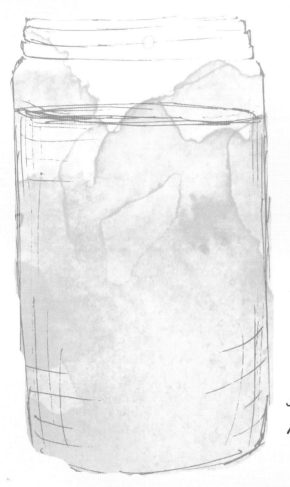

Green Smoothie Recipe

*8 oz spinach
*1 Tbsp almond butter
*1 Tbsp coconut oil
*1 banana
*1 cup frozen
  blueberries

↑

This is super healthy and super easy. Great way to get nutrients in your body quick!

YOU KNOW WHAT'S HEALTHIER THAN KALE?

Loving your body.

lochia

/ˈlōkēə, ˈläk-/

noun

1. The normal discharge from the uterus after childbirth.

   "It's been 6 weeks...When will this lochia end!?"

Drink water and
get some sun.
You're basically a
houseplant with
more complicated
emotions.

Hopefully you won't need this!

Try to pee,

then fart,

and then poop.

As soon as you can!

ON C-SECTIONS

RECOVERY TIPS

- Walk as soon as you can—it really helps with the crazy swelling that will happen post-surgery.

- Make someone bring you green juices every morning. (You need some nutrients, and hospital food ain't cutting it.)

- The opioid-based painkillers cause constipation. Get off them ASAP.

Females are strong as hell.

Vaginal Birth Recovery Tips

Peeing, pooping, and toilet paper (not to mention sex) may be terrifying for a while, but here are a few tips to give you some relief down there:

*Sitz (German for "seat") bath—you can DIY with Epsom salts and essential oils, or just using plain warm water will feel good too!

*Pads soaked in witch hazel + water, and then frozen.

*Numbing sprays, like Dermoplast.

*When peeing, use a peri bottle with warm water.

*Donut pillows—because sitting may hurt for a while.

POOPING DURING DELIVERY IS ACTUALLY A GOOD THING!

↑

Firstly, it means that you were pushing correctly. Second, it helps your babe develop their microbiome, which is essential for a lifetime of health.

Embrace Granny Panties

Stock up, because these big undies keep the big pads you'll need to wear in place. Another fun option: buy adult diaper-style underwear so you don't have to worry about any shifting pads!

Night Sweats

Yup, this is a thing. It can last up to 8 weeks as your body gets rid of all that extra fluid it needed for baby.

Gas and Constipation

Whether you had a vaginal delivery or a C-section, the prospect of pooping can be daunting (if not downright terrifying), and you can get backed up! Do yourself a favor and stock up on dried apricots or prunes to help get things easing along.

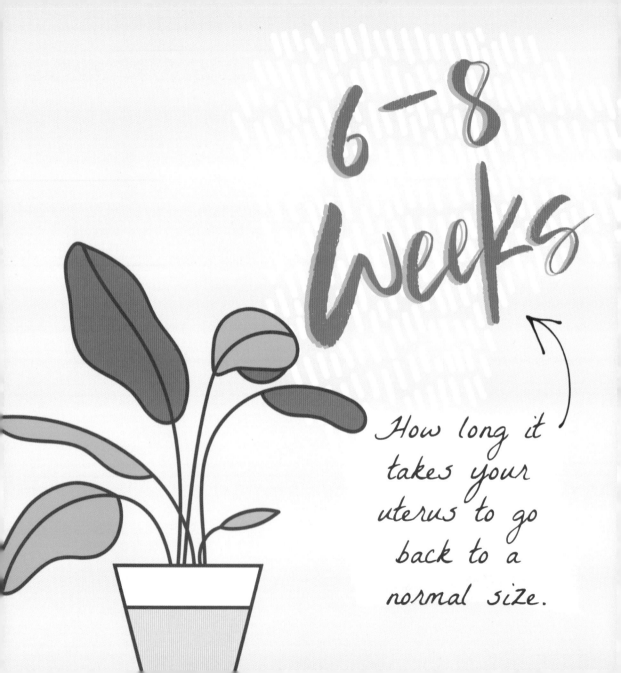

6-8 weeks

How long it takes your uterus to go back to a normal size.

YOUR BODY IS SO AMAZING AND MAGICAL AND HAS CREATED LIFE. LOVE AND RESPECT IT.

Little by
little, one
travels far.

JRR Tolkien

Remember, your body has been stretching
and adjusting 9 months long. Give it at
least that much time to get back to normal.

self-care

/self'ker/

noun

1. The practice of taking actions to preserve one's own health.

   "My self-care regimen includes a morning green smoothie and an Epsom salt lavender bath at night."

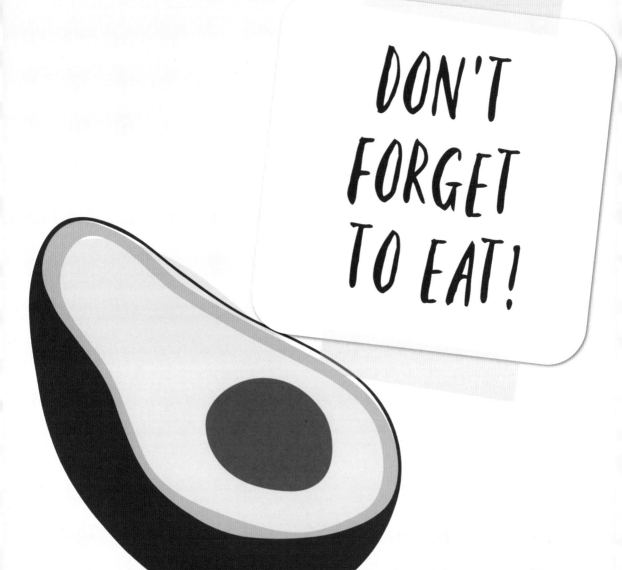

But seriously, don't forget to eat. This actually happens all the time and your body is working so, so hard; you need to care for it.

Remember your air mask!

WAYS TO BEEF UP YOUR IMMUNE SYSTEM:

* Garlic tea.
* Take Zinc.
* Drink lots of water and green juice.
* Sleep more, if you can.

GARLIC TEA:

* Half a lemon, squeezed (save the juice)
* 1-2 cloves minced garlic
* ½ tsp cayenne pepper
* 1 Tbsp honey

Combine in a mug and pour boiling water on top.

POSTURE IS MY CARDIO

This is actually a legit workout. Try to remind yourself while walking the stroller or cooking in the kitchen. It's a full-body workout you can do anytime.

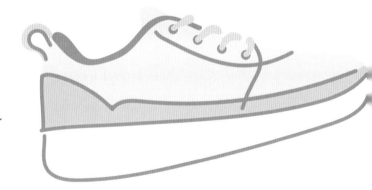

DANCER POSTURE

Instructions:

*Try to be as vertical as possible.

*Engage abs: tummy should feel tight, pulled up, and in.

*Tuck your bottom and flatten your back.

*Pull shoulders back and down, widening them.

Keep going, no matter what.

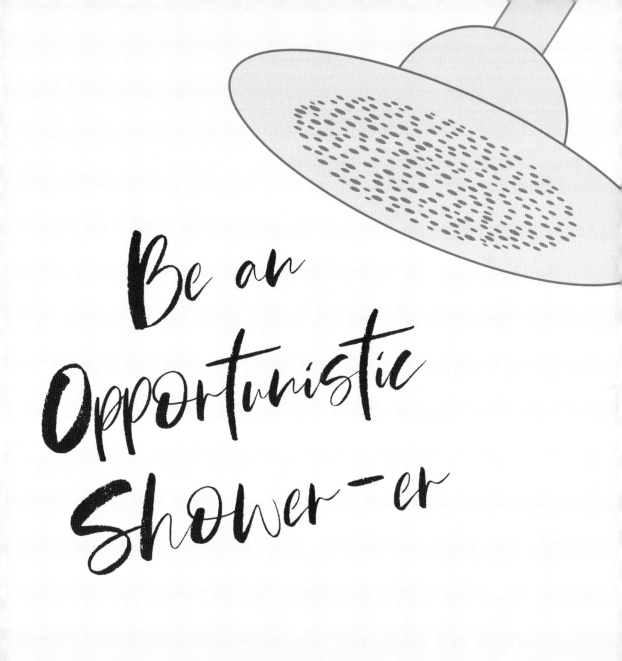

Be an
Opportunistic
Shower-er

Girl, you already have what it takes.

Live,

Laugh,

Wear

Sunscreen

WHEN IN DOUBT

DANCE IT OUT

A good laugh and a long sleep are the two best cures for anything.

Irish Proverb

PROTECT YOUR ENERGY

My mission in life is not merely to survive, but to thrive; and to do so with some passion, some compassion, some humor, and some style.

Maya Angelou

CHAPTER 6

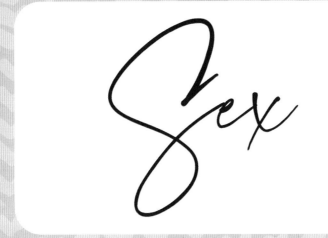

Sex, I'm not gonna lie, I'm a big fan. In the midst of the rollercoaster of hormones you are on, the ones you get as a result of loving sex have a great normalizing effect. After sex, I generally feel calmer, clear-eyed, happier, and more in control. That said, you have just experienced the eventual consequence of having sex (i.e., being pregnant and going through childbirth), so you are viscerally aware of that consequence...and it's scary. Not to mention, your body went through A LOT to get that baby out. Your body may not be physically ready for sex for a while, and you should honor that. Between scars, tears, and a deflated tummy, it may be hard to even recognize your own body, let alone feel sexy in it. My advice is to practice so much self love, it's silly. Love your amazing body, and love your amazing partner—you created life together! Honor your body's timeline & trust your libido. She knows the way.

FIRST OF ALL,
YOU'RE REALLY PRETTY.

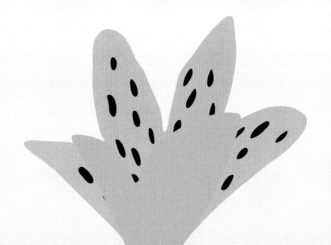

RULE # 1
NO SEX FOR 6 WEEKS!

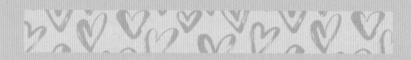

RULE #2
USE PROTECTION

Back-to-back pregnancies are gnarly on your body!

Give
yourself
time.

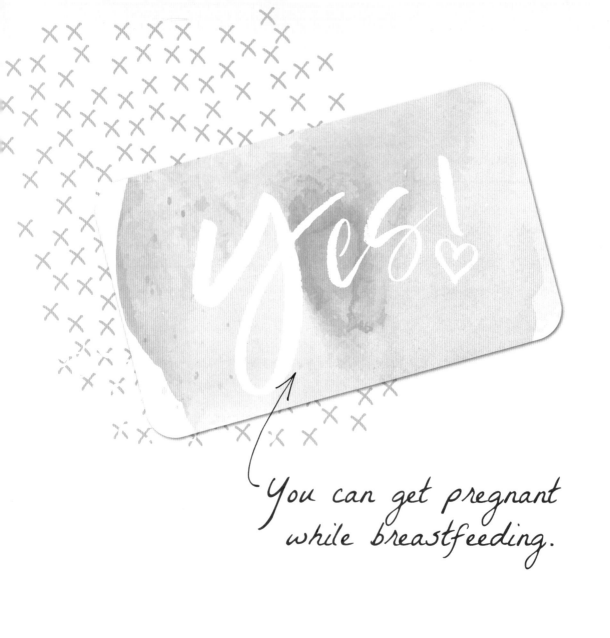

yes! ♡

You can get pregnant
while breastfeeding.

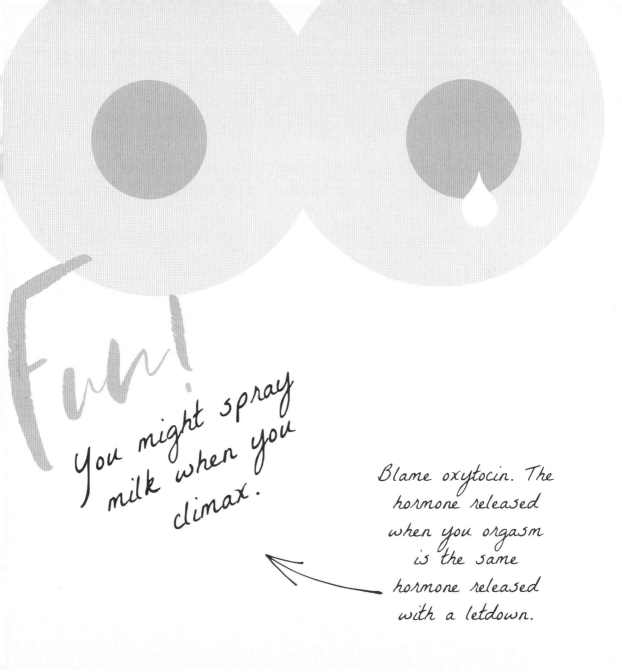

Fun!

You might spray milk when you climax.

Blame oxytocin. The hormone released when you orgasm is the same hormone released with a letdown.

Make it fun!

YOUR NEW BEST FRIEND:

LUBE

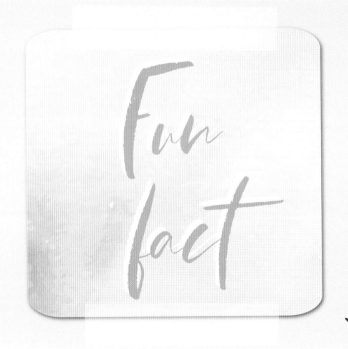

In the first few months after baby, the hormones are similar to menopause. It makes sense you aren't into it yet, and that's OK.

THERE'S NO NEED TO RUSH; SOAK UP EVERY MOMENT.

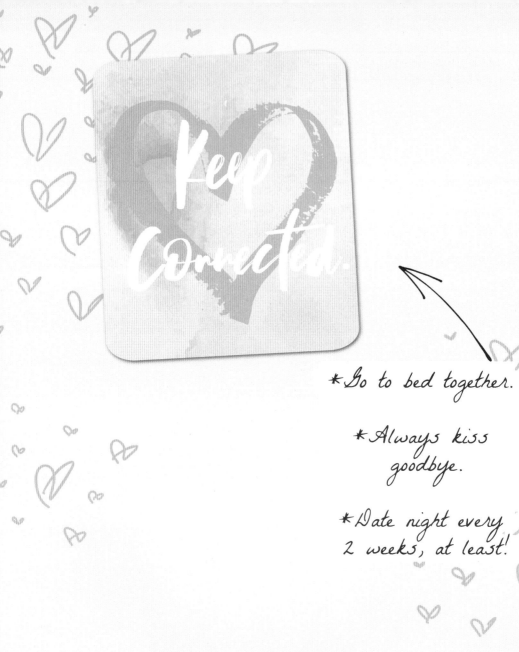

*Go to bed together.

*Always kiss goodbye.

*Date night every 2 weeks, at least!

YOUR PARTNER'S WAY IS DIFFERENT, BUT NOT WRONG.

Once you are a mom, you sort of become a control freak (at least I did), and nobody handles your baby exactly as you would. Try to be self-aware about it and focus on how amazing it is to have a partner who loves your baby so much and wants to help!

EVOKE THE 2 HOUR NO-TALKING RULE

Nikki Lovett

Sometimes it really helps to give each other a minute. Sleep deprivation and fluctuating hormones can be a lethal combination to civil discourse. You love your partner, and they love your baby; take a breath and decide to talk about it later.

YOU ARE
EXACTLY
WHERE
YOU NEED
TO BE.

YOU GLOW GIRL

and you are sexy as hell!

Darling,
you are
so fine.

CHAPTER 7

Baby

Awwwww babies—those perfect tiny toes, that perfect little nose, and their sweet new smiles make all the exhaustion worth it somehow. Babies can't care for themselves, so they require a lot of time and effort. You need to keep them clean, keep them fed, and make sure they are sleeping enough—it's draining! Babies don't have too many options in how they communicate all their needs, so it's a lot of crying at first. It makes sense; it's all they've got. Which means your job becomes a big game of "decode the cry," which can be very frustrating. As always, don't beat yourself up—you are doing your best. Every baby is different: some cry less, some cry more, some like things certain ways. Your baby will definitely throw you some curveballs, and normally right when you think you have things figured out. Try to roll with it and keep finding solace in those gorgeous little eyes. You got this, mama!!

T R U S T
Y O U R
G U T

If something seems off or wrong, trust your gut and talk to your doctor.

BABIES LOVE SUNSHINE

And so does their booty. Get that booty some sunshine and you can avoid diaper rash or get rid of it!

CLEAR UP DIAPER RASH FAST:

SUNSHINE

+

AIR

+

ZINC OXIDE

CREAM

CRYING PEAKS AT 6 WEEKS

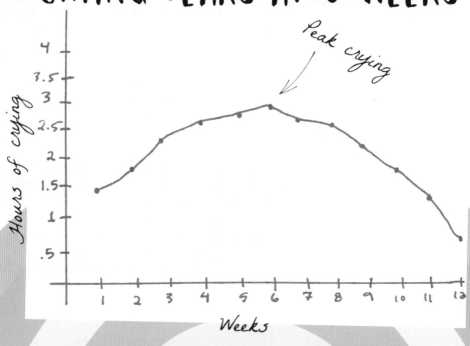

Peak crying

Hours of crying

Weeks

Babies cry to
release stress,
just like you.

TROUBLESHOOTING A CRYING BABY

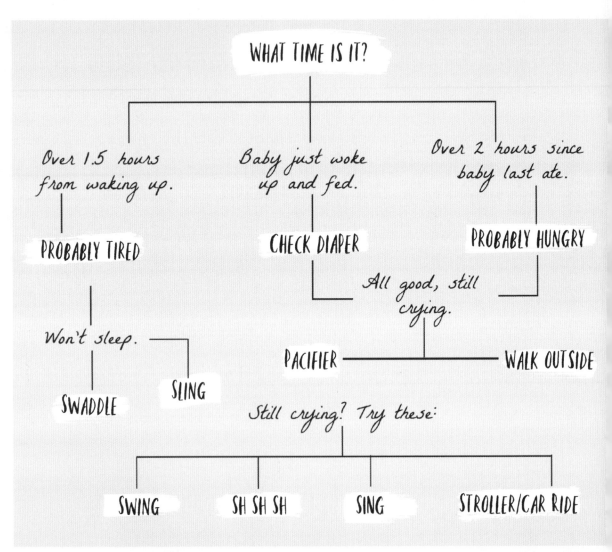

WHAT TIME IS IT?

Over 1.5 hours from waking up. → PROBABLY TIRED

Baby just woke up and fed. → CHECK DIAPER

Over 2 hours since baby last ate. → PROBABLY HUNGRY

PROBABLY TIRED

Won't sleep. → SWADDLE / SLING

All good, still crying.

PACIFIER —— WALK OUTSIDE

Still crying? Try these:

SWING   SH SH SH   SING   STROLLER/CAR RIDE

When your baby won't
stop crying, remember:

*Crying is good for
their lungs.

*Crying is cardio for
babies.

*Crying is how babies
release stress.

colic

/col·ic/

noun

1. Persistent, prolonged period of intense crying
   each day.

   "This baby has been crying for hours and is
   absolutely inconsolable. I think he may have
   colic. Let's call the doctor."

OK mama, just breathe. This is a
hard one, but you will get through it.
You and baby will be OK.

ON COLIC:

* 1 in 5 babies develop colic.

* Usually occurs between weeks 2 and 4.

* Placing your baby in a safe place like their crib to take a break is a good idea.

*This is very hard, but it does pass.

If your baby cries inconsolably for 3 hours or more a day, consider talking to your doctor about the possibility of colic and how to treat it.

Expect baby's first "true" smile at 6-12 weeks.

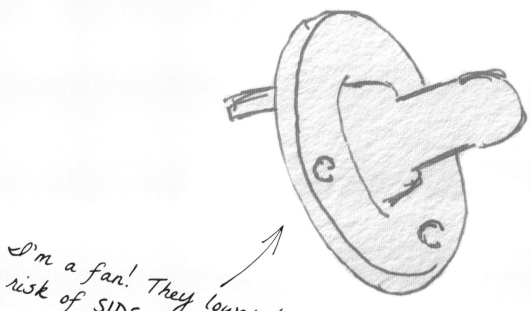

I'm a fan! They lower the risk of SIDS and soothe a stressed-out baby!

BABIES GET SICK 3-9 TIMES IN THEIR FIRST YEAR.

Top 5 Reasons for Doctor Visits
in the First Year:

(in no particular order)

* Sleep struggles
* Gas, fussiness, feeding/breastfeeding issues
* Fevers
* Management of colds/coughs
* "Baby blues" (postpartum depression)

RECORD STUFF ON YOUR PHONE!

You will be amazed just how much your memory sucks when you are sleep deprived. Use your phone to write down questions for your doctor, record unusual behaviors, or anything else you don't want to forget!

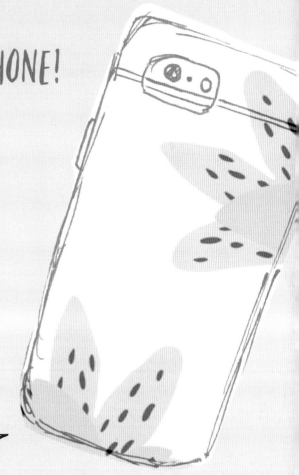

AVERAGE SLEEP NEEDS BY AGE

Age	Total per day	# of naps
>2 months	16-20 hours	4+
3 months	15-18 hours	4
4 months	14-15 hours	3-4
5 months	14-15 hours	3
6 months	14-15 hours	2-3
7 months	14 hours	2-3
8 months	14 hours	2-3
9 months	14 hours	2
10 months	14 hours	2
11 months	13-14 hours	2
12 months	13-14 hours	1-2

*Remember these are averages.

SLINGS & CARRIERS REDUCE CRYING!

Baby-wearing for 3 hours a day reduces overall crying by 43%.

witching hour
/ˈwiCHiNG - ˈou(ə)r/

noun

1. The normal fussy period that most babies experience anytime between 4pm and 12am. This normally starts at 2–3 weeks and resolves by 3–4 months.

   "My normally happy baby becomes inconsolable during his 5:00 pm witching hour every night—make it stop!"

This too shall pass, but it's exhausting while it happens.

BEWARE OF OVERSTIMLATION

When babies get overstimulated, they
will get fussy and cry. It's pretty
easy to overstimulate a baby,
especially in the first 3 months.
Babies can't block out bright lights
and loud noises. Taking them to a
quiet, dark room can help calm them
down.

*Clean everything with vinegar.

Keep it Simple

*Coconut oil for cradle cap, dry skin, and pain-free Band-Aid removal.

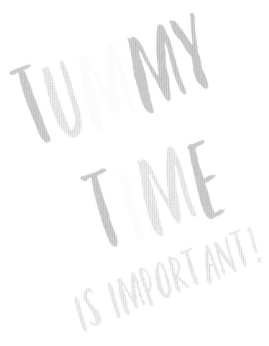

TUMMY TIME IS IMPORTANT!

* Full-term babies can do it right away.

* Start with 2-3 minute chunks.

* By 3-4 months, you want to be doing it 20-30 minutes a day.

* Strengthens neck muscles.

* Promotes head control.

* Builds muscles for rolling and eventually crawling.

Every little movement helps, but if your babe is too frustrated, take a break.

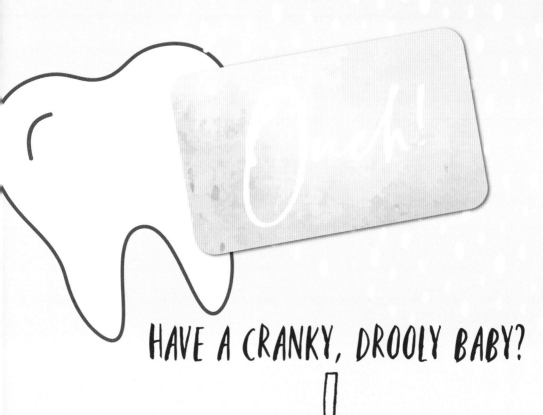

HAVE A CRANKY, DROOLY BABY?

⬇

It's probably teething.

Good to know:

-Teething pain comes before tooth eruption.

-First tooth normally erupts around 6 months, but there is huge variability in when teeth come in (3-12 months.)

-Front teeth come first.

Teething isn't always a big deal, and most of the time teething doesn't really hurt. But sometimes it does, so here are a few things that help:

-Massaging sore, swollen gums with your finger.

-Freeze things and let the baby chew on them (i.e., washcloths, chew toys, cucumber rings, bagels).

- Tylenol* if they are really, really miserable. (I only needed this when molars came in.)

*Ask your doctor for the correct dosage of Tylenol.

BABY PROOFING

=

STRESSING LESS

Let your baby roam
(at least in your home).

BABY'S

Perfect

FIRST FOOD

AVOCADOS!

SOLID FOOD

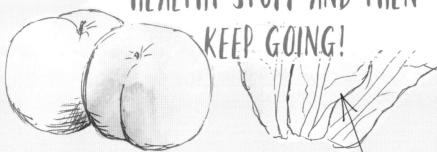

BABIES WILL TRY ALMOST ANYTHING, SO START WITH HEALTHY STUFF AND THEN KEEP GOING!

It's only "gross" to them when they are older because it's not normal.

BABY SIGN LANGUAGE

More

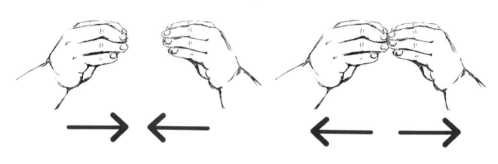

All done

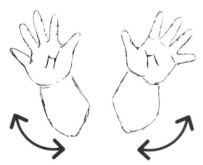 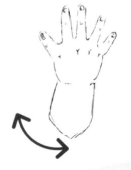 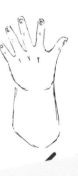

I used these 2 the most!

BABY SIGN LANGUAGE

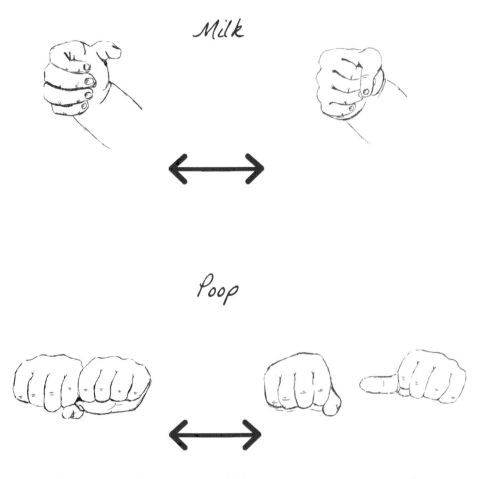

Milk

Poop

It doesn't feel real at first, and then it feels really real too fast. On the hard days and moments, lean on gratitude; on the good ones, relish. Savor all the snuggles, even in the middle of the night, because these little ones grow so fast. Soon those smiles and cries become small words and then conversations. Be prepared to be amazed every step of the way. Being a mom is truly one of life's greatest treasures, and you were made for this. You got this, Mama.

♡

Liz

This book is dedicated to the enormous love between all best friends.

Acknowledgments:

Katie, I love you so much and don't know how I would survive being a mom without you. From peeing our pants laughing about crazy things our kids do, to crying when we are so tired it hurts, you are my inspiration always. Truman, Hendrik, and Escher, I didn't know love until I loved you; thank you for bringing me more joy than I ever thought possible. My perfect partner, Casey, what an amazing life we have created; I am grateful every day for you. My village, Gamma, Grandpa Ocean, Grandma and Grandpa Swenson, all the uncles, aunties, cousins, and mom-friends, thank you for keeping me sane. I am such a better mom because of you.

About the Author

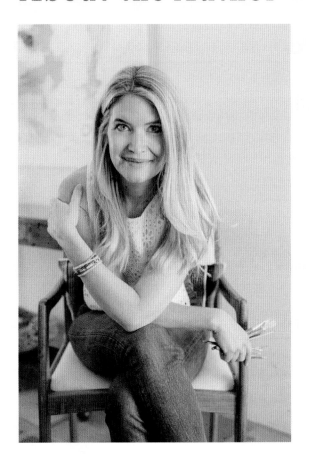

LIZ SWENSON

is a high school math teacher with a master's in Mathematics. She is an author, illustrator, and painter living in San Clemente, California, with her husband and 3 perfect children.

About Familius

Visit Our Website: www.familius.com

Familius is a global trade publishing company that publishes books and other content to help families be happy. We believe that the family is the fundamental unit of society and that happy families are the foundation of a happy life. We recognize that every family looks different, and we passionately believe in helping all families find greater joy. To that end, we publish books for children and adults that invite families to live the Familius Nine Habits of Happy Family Life: love together, play together, learn together, work together, talk together, heal together, read together, eat together, and laugh together.

Founded in 2012, Familius is located in Sanger, California.

Connect

Facebook: www.facebook.com/paterfamilius

Twitter: @familiustalk, @paterfamilius1

Pinterest: www.pinterest.com/familius

Instagram: @familiustalk

FAMILIUS

"The most important work you ever do will be within the walls of your own home."

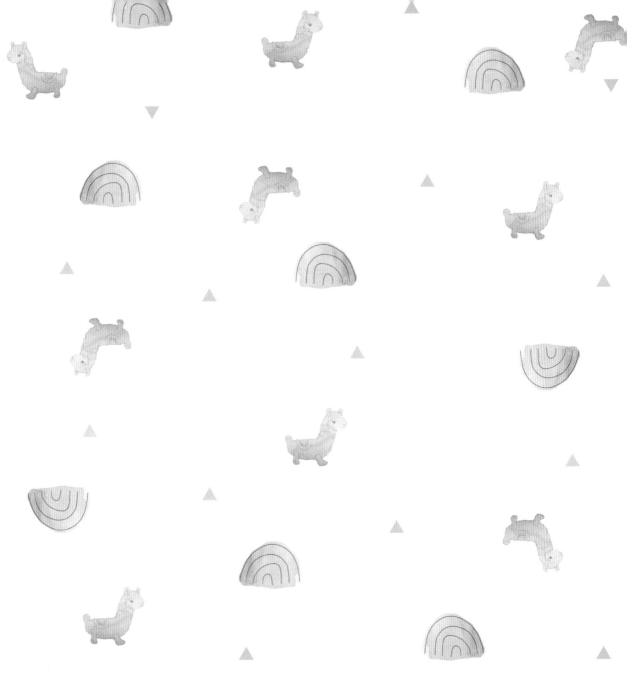

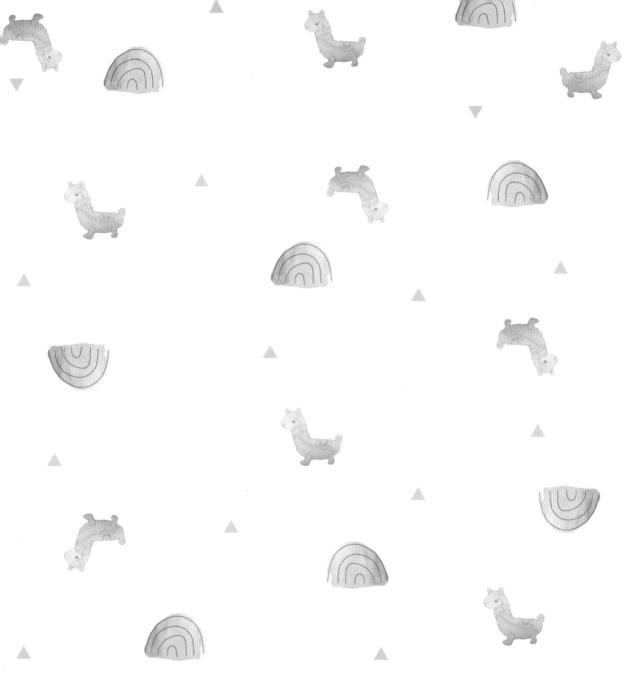